I0776189

Just Say Sometimes

Healthy Appetites for
Unrepressed Souls

Volume Two, Testaments of the
Temple of the Circus Monkey

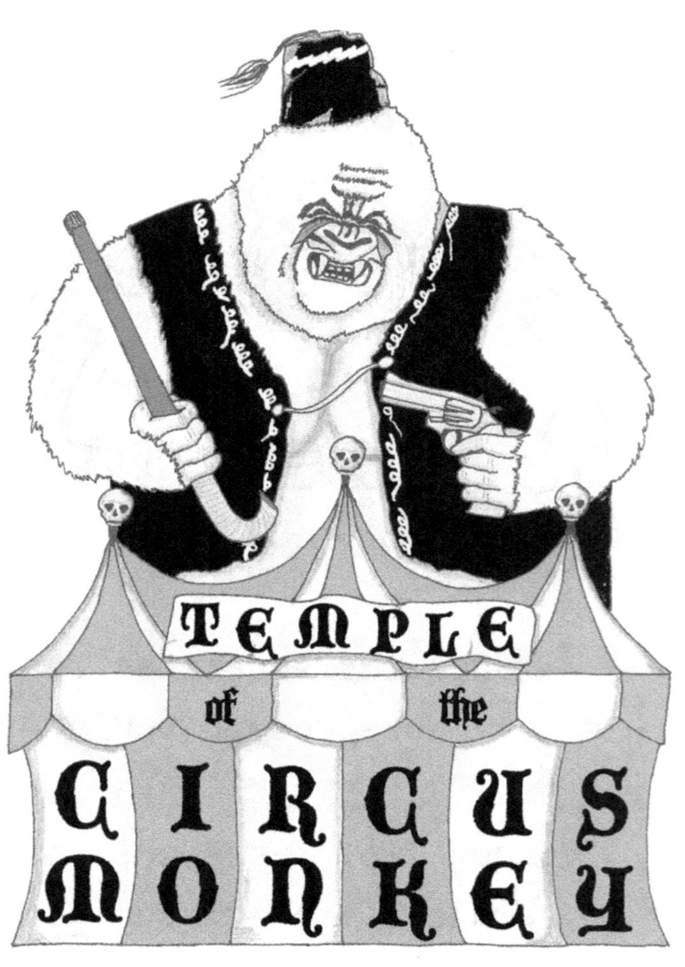

Just Say Sometimes, 2nd Edition is published
by the Temple of the Circus Monkey.
All opinions are those of the Author,
Archbishop Angus McIntosh.
All rights reserved.
Permission inquiries Angus@kwchop.org
The year 2017 of the Common Era
Nevada, USA, Earth

Enter
at your
own
risk

A READER'S GUIDE

Before you enter into my world there are a few things I think we should get straight. First of all, I'm an adult and I use colorful language. By that I mean words like "fuck." If you're offended by adult language please go find something written for children. I also tend to use a stream of consciousness style that can take some getting used to. I'm sure you'll work it out.

Since you're reading this I assume that you're serious about taking control of your life. I want to make it perfectly clear that I DON'T CARE what you decide to do. I only care that you get to make the choice yourself and take responsibility for the ramifications. Most likely you'll find different answers than I did. Good for you. Find your own joy and fun.

I expect that most readers will ignore some parts of each book. That's cool. If you already have a strong personal philosophy or religion you should feel free to discard mine. The skills I've presented will work just as well for you anyway. Use what you can and ignore the rest. My ego won't be offended.

Readers will quickly discover that I tend to ignore the social taboos against discussing things like spirituality and sex. It's disconcerting to some people that I talk openly about faith and God. Sorry, but they're a big part of life whether you talk about them or not. Before you start I want to make my own views perfectly clear. I doubt that there's a big anthropomorphic god. I think there is some universal spirit or energy that informs our lives and if you want to call it god, go right ahead.

Regardless of religion I believe in Joy and fun, beauty and love, compassion and kindness. We are all free, but only the strong willed can exercise that freedom in a world full of bitter squirrels and demons. These books are the method I use to center myself, feel good, and find joy. I hope the ideas in them help you too. Just remember, as Shakespeare said, "There are more things on heaven and earth, Horatio, than are dreamt of in your philosophy."

10

Just Say Sometimes

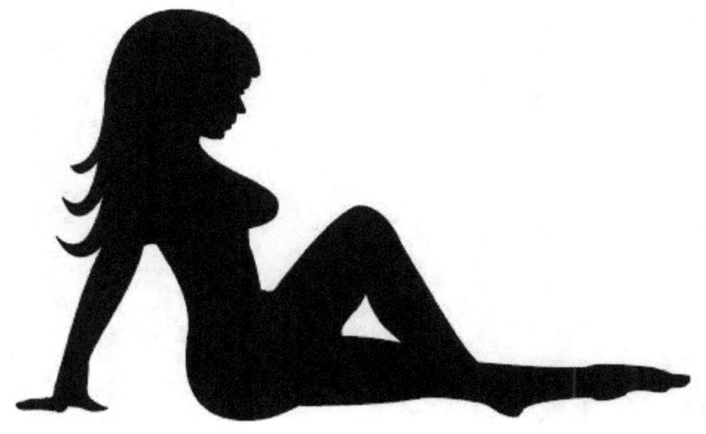

Angus McIntosh

Archbishop of the

Temple of the Circus Monkey

All illustrations by Amanda McIntosh

This book is dedicated to every cute
girl I ever ogled. Thanks for
everything.

Table of Contents

CHAPTER ONE: IT'S TIME TO ACT

Just what the world needs, another fucking diet book. Well, not exactly. How about a little clarity instead? How about a book that deals with all of your appetites and not just your culinary ones? How about a book that stops blaming people for genetics? How about a book that acknowledges that eating is good fun and shouldn't be used to shame? How about we leave political causes, profit motives and hateful world views out and replace them with facts and a little joy? How about we stop talking about our "feelings" about food and start talking about our actions? Wouldn't that be a little different?

Oh yeah, actions. You remember those, don't you? They're what we used to take before we started to navel gaze and ruminate and argue. If you want to listen to a bunch of bullshit about how you're fat because of your inner child or evil crap peddlers at McDonald's or your own laziness than you need to head your fat ass back out to the bookstore and buy one of the ten thousand diet books that will cater to your self indulgent non action.

For the very few of you that
continue, we need to get a couple of
things straight. First of all, I'm
kind of fat. And I like it. I'm
5'9" and weigh around 200 pounds. I
also have black belts and medals for
finishing marathons. A few years
back while developing this diet I
got down to a very svelte 155 pounds
and I was miserable. My body wanted
more weight. So I put back on 50
pounds. On purpose. I like my big
belly and it likes me. Get over it.

The next thing you need to do
is check out the table of contents.
How many chapters in this book
actually cover the diet? That's
right, two. Chapters 6 and 10.
That's because diets are really
fucking simple and two chapters are
more than enough. The rest of the
chapters cover your other appetites
and try to shed a little light on
the giant clusterfuck that is the
food and diet industry in the United
States. Read the whole thing though
because you'll need all the
information at some point. Besides,
I took the time to write it and you
bought the book, so you might as
well.

Speaking of that, why did you
buy this book? (Thanks, by the way.

I need the money and the ego
gratification.) Are you fat?
Unhealthy? Unhappy in your body?
Take a few minutes and get clear
about your motivations. It will
help. Anyway, I'm going to assume
that you bought it because something
is wrong with your life and your
instinct says that your diet or
appetites are at least partially to
blame. You might be right, and even
if you're wrong you might be right,
too.

I'll try to be a little less
confusing. Your appetites might in
fact be a big part of your problem.
You might actually be an unhealthy
fat pig. If so, this book can help.
On the other hand, you might be
absolutely fine and just think
you're a fat unhealthy pig. In
which case this book is still going
to help. Why? Because clearing up
that little misunderstanding will
give you a handle on personal
responsibility and that might go a
long way to curing the real source
of your dissatisfaction. How cool
is that?

How is that possible? Why is a
spiritual revolutionary writing a
diet book? Same answer. In order
to change the world we need to first
change ourselves. Trite, but true.

The basis of revolution is the magic combination of freedom, power, and control. These things give you CHOICES and that, my friends, is something we all need to practice. What better place to practice choices than your own body and its appetites?

As you may know, this book is part of a series. I would strongly suggest checking out a couple of the other books, as well as this one. "Enough Already" is a good choice if you want to understand change and motivation a little better. If you've failed at other diets, I'd definitely suggest forking over the cash. "Get Off Your Ass" is the exercise companion workout to this book. Exercise and diet complement each other. Attacking the issue of bodily control on two fronts simultaneously just makes sense. If you work out, you're more likely to make good diet choices and vice versa. Besides, there's nothing worse than losing weight and finding flabby muscles underneath. "Inner Workout Fu" adds a spiritual dimension and teaches you a new way to understand your body. All three are available through the web site. Check out the end of the book for details.

The last thing you need to know
is that I LIKE appetites. I adore
rich food, whisky, cigars, ice
cream, and Coca-Cola. I love sex
and cute girls. If you're looking
for someone to toe the politically
correct line and tell you that these
things are bad you are really in the
wrong book. I don't believe that
and I won't tolerate the attitude.
If anything this book is more likely
to help you enjoy those things MORE,
not less. Not exactly a normal diet
book.

Your body is good. So are its
appetites. You just need to
exercise control and make decent,
informed choices. If you can't
change your diet, how can you change
the world? If you can't find joy in
your appetites, how will you ever
create joy in the universe? You
can't. So let's get started…

CHAPTER 2: APPETITES AND ALIBIS

"He was a man of vast and varied appetites." Look at that phrase. Consider it deeply. In your mind is that a compliment or a condemnation? That's a good question and the answer will go a long way toward teaching you something about yourself. The more you're pleased by that statement the higher your capacity for joy is likely to be. If you're threatened by it you should give joy some serious thought because appetites are good, natural parts of our human experience.

Appetites encompass everything that goes into or comes out of our bodies. They're the way our body interacts with the world around us, affecting our moods, our ideals, our economies, our relationships, and even our body chemistry. Fulfilling them provides our strongest motivations and in them we find the roots of war as well as the epiphanies of love. They provide the path to both ecstasy and hell. That's why every religion in history has sought to control them and every repressed fucktard has tried to suppress them. You cannot hope to find joy or freedom or change without understanding, embracing, and controlling your appetites. Avoiding this responsibility is just creating alibis for your own complacency.

In this book I've broken appetites into three categories: diet, sex, and inebriation. Food is the most obvious appetite. We get hungry and need nourishment so we put things in our mouth and swallow them. Sex is pretty self-explanatory, too. Our genes want to survive through time so they push us to replicate. Inebriation might surprise you, but it's an appetite just as surely as the previous two. Our brains crave experiences and just love to alter their own state. Inebriation affects many of the same areas as sex and food, just a little more directly. If you want to change your life, you need to get control of all three. By the way, control does not abstention. It means conscious choice.

I can already hear the complaints. "That might be too hard." "Can't I just start with one and maybe get to the others a little later?" "I just want to lose a little weight, why do I have to deal

with sex?" Shut the fuck up. Do
you want real change? Do you want
to deal with this shit ONCE AND FOR
ALL? Well then you have to do all
three at once. Unless, of course,
you're clinically schizophrenic.
     You're one person. You have
one set of skills and your own
unique style of handling the world.
That is as it should be. It also
means that on some level you're
going to deal with all of your
appetites in exactly the same way.
For any new skill to be effective it
had better work equally well for all
three. Otherwise, you'll sabotage
yourself and eventually fail. I'm
telling you the truth whether you
like it or not.
     Let's use some examples.
Lucretia wants to lose a few pounds
so she goes to the bookstore and
chooses a diet book. She follows
the diet and successfully drops the
weight. But Lucretia is still
unfulfilled and sexually repressed.
So she begins to resort back to ice
cream in order to fill that hole.
And the weight comes back. Ignatius
knows he needs to cut down his
weight because the cardiologist said
he was gonna die soon if he didn't.
So he goes on a diet but he doesn't
lose much weight or get any

healthier because he still gets drunk and smokes pot every day. Duh.

Still not convinced? Still don't think they're so connected? Think about it. A rich meal isn't really complete without a glass of wine. Smoking a little pot makes you hungry as hell. Food and sex have a lot in common. And we all know that sexual inhibitions drop with the addition of inebriates. That's why we get girls drunk! So drop your resistance, address all three appetites and quit bellyaching. "It's too hard" is a weak ass alibi.

Every creature on earth has the same appetites as you do. Every tiger, turtle, and tsetse fly wants to eat, fuck, and mellow out a little. Infants come out of the womb looking for their first meal and at puberty the instinct to get laid and stoned hits like a typhoon. Adult humans are different than turtles, tots, and teens. We have a better skillset and more perspective, or at least we should. That's what makes choices and growth possible.

As an adult you should have developed a sense of self awareness, some sense of who you are and what

you're doing. You have the
perspective of time so you can plan
for the future. You understand the
concept of delayed gratification
even if you don't like it. You
probably even have a pretty good
grasp of cause and effect. If I eat
this, that will happen. You can say
the words "I want," "no," and
"later." Or at least I hope you
can.

If you put all this skill and
awareness together you get choice.
Once you make choices you can begin
to affect change. If you want more
help with this I suggest you read
"Enough Already." The more choices
you make, the more control you have
over your appetites. The more
control you exert, the more likely
you are to find joy and health.
Having control is what
differentiates adults from children
and humans from animals. Conceding
choice and control makes you an
infant or animal and that's a pretty
lame alibi.

Speaking of lame alibis, let's
discuss scapegoating. The way you
deal with your appetites is your
responsibility. End of story.
Therapy might reveal why you have
bad habits. Religion might explain
why you're repressed. Crappy

abusive parents suck. I know all about that. How you got fucked up might well be somebody else's fault but not fixing it is yours. You're an adult now and only you can control yourself. Forget about how you got here and move on or you're destined to live with the damage for the rest of your life.

Perhaps the lamest alibi is "I'll let someone else do it." People who can't handle the responsibility for their own appetites set up elaborate external controls instead of the more effective internal ones used by adult humans. They call these external controls things like "God's word" and "the Law." It's a simple formula. I can't keep from being a drug addict, so I'll make it illegal to take drugs. I can't control where I put my dick, so I'll decide that God hates sex. What a crock. They assume that just because they're too fucking weak to handle life that no one else can do it either. If someone complains, they lock them up or stone them or start whining about protecting the children. That's very close to my definition of evil and a shitty excuse for a human being. Don't let yourself fall prey to this brand of alibis. They start from the totally wrong premise that appetites are bad and need to be repressed.

Appetites are good. You exist today because of them. If your ancestors didn't fuck, you clearly wouldn't be here. All of the people who couldn't store fat died off when times got hard. Inebriation was undoubtedly the moving force behind many of the inventions and artwork that make life better today. Trying to suppress your appetites is like trying to stop getting taller as a kid or trying to stop sleeping ever again. You just can't do it and it's stupid to try.

Besides being pointless, appetite repression is a sure way to kill joy. As I said earlier, appetites are how we experience the world around us. If you want to live a full life you need to sample what the planet has to offer. Food is wonderful. Getting drunk or stoned is really fun. Sex is great. Why would that be the case if God or Evolution didn't want us to experience them? That makes no fucking sense. Demonizing appetites is the weakest alibi of all.

Having said that, let's not get carried away. Letting our appetites run rampant isn't such a good idea

either. (In fact, just giving
ourselves over to our appetites is
just another bullshit way to keep
from taking responsibility.) Our
bodies are fairly tightly regulated
little machines and too much of some
appetites will throw us way out of
balance. A dead body is pretty
useless so some compromises must be
made. The object of control, and
this book, is to help you find the
right combination of control and
indulgence to keep you both healthy
and joyful.

CHAPTER 3: BALANCING FUN AND HEALTH

"Everything in moderation, especially moderation." That's what my grandfather used to say. No, really, he did. And that old Scottish son of a bitch was exactly right. He even practiced what he preached. He wasn't a smoker because it might have interfered with his responsibilities. The day he retired he went out and bought a pack of cigarettes. He figured that he was now free to indulge and that whatever damage they might cause would be slight since he was already seventy. He smoked happily the last few years of his life and loved every fucking second of it.

While I appreciate his tactics I'm not willing to wait until I'm seventy to have a little fun. Therefore I needed to figure out how to apply his moderation dictum a little differently. Especially the part about being moderate in moderation. That particular journey led to this book.

I wanted to know how to balance my appetites so that I could have a lot of fun and still be reasonably healthy. Achieving that balance is

the trick to long term success. Too
much healthy and you're deprived of
joy. Too much bad food and
inebriates and you might die young
or at least have a crappy old age.
Finding your own balance is the task
before you and I hope this book
helps you do that.

Chapters four through seven
will explain the forces working
against you and give you a few
simple rules about food and your
genetic destiny. You live in a
particular society at a particular
time and you need to know how that
affects your chances for success.
Forewarned is forearmed.

Chapters eight and ten will
give you a chance to clean the slate
and define your most efficient diet.
Take note, I said most efficient
diet, not what you have to do. Once
you've determined your proper diet
you have the freedom to ignore it
whenever you want. Life is full of
opportunities to misbehave and you
shouldn't deprive yourself of that
delicious feeling that can only be
gained by doing something naughty.

Since you have power of choice
you can develop the confidence to
make really bad short-term decisions
in the name of pleasure and know
that you'll return to your healthier

choices when that's appropriate. Of course bad choices have consequences, but you'll know what they are so you can at least make an informed decision. It's analogous to being offered one more drink when you know you've really had enough. Most of the time you'll decide to pass up the drink in favor of a hangover free morning but sometimes you'll say "screw it" and have three more drinks. You know what the pleasure will cost, and you're willing to pay it. Knowledge is power but not necessarily wisdom.

Chapters eleven and twelve cover sex, drugs, and rock & roll. They offer realistic advice about these societally touchy subjects. As I keep saying, you need to get a handle on all three appetites to have any hope of finding that elusive balance.

I can't even begin to explain how crucially important balancing your appetites between joy and health is to your destiny. The quality of your intellect, your emotional world, and your spiritual life depend completely on both sides of the equation. Good health makes you smarter, happier and more open to the spirit. Joy makes your life worth living and enhances every

other quality. Any diet and all
your choices should strive to
maximize BOTH of these things. Of
course the world doesn't necessarily
want you to do that...

CHAPTER 4: BEWARE THE NEW PURITANS

There's a great early episode of South Park where my hero Eric Cartman complains of how everything that day involved something going into or out of his ass. I think that perfectly sums up the busybody puritans who fuck up this country on a daily basis. Rather than pay attention to their own sorry lives they constantly concern themselves with everything that goes into or out of someone else's body or what everyone else is doing with their genitals.

Taking control of your appetites is hard. If it were simple we'd all have done it by now. Balancing health and joy is complicated. Delayed gratification sucks. Discipline and motivation take tremendous strength and courage. In many ways you'll find that you end up working against yourself or sabotaging your own efforts. But no, that's not enough. Some repressed fuckhead has to pile shame and guilt onto your psyche, too. It's a damn nuisance but in order to take control of YOUR OWN appetites you first have to weed out their malevolent influence.

So who are these trolls? As you might remember from elementary school, the puritans (I refuse to capitalize such a shitty word) were some of the first white people to colonize North America. Seems they were too damn wacky for England so they fled to the New World in order to create their own joyless religious utopia. Even though those fuckers are long dead, their dreary world view became part of the basic fabric of who we are as Americans. While I admire both their hardiness and their commitment to their belief system was a complete mess and it continues to make the world a more miserable place than it needs to be.

The puritan conception of God was pretty simple; if you like something, God hates it. They took the Bible pretty literally. Women were responsible for the fall from grace and had to be subjugated. The devil tempted you constantly with pleasures of the flesh and if you succumbed, it was proof that God had already condemned you to hell. Proving you were a good person and predestined for heaven meant denying yourself the enjoyment of good food, good drink, and good sex. In fact the work "puritan" comes from the

belief that other churches were too
tolerant or lax.

     Everything about their society
was anti-freedom. Strict and severe
interpretation of the Bible.
Proving your predestination to
heaven through constant hard labor.
Unquestioning subservience to father
and town elders. Evangelical work
to convert or conquer anyone with a
different world view. A complete
lack of tolerance for individuality.
I can't imagine a philosophy that
would allow less joy.

     It's not hard now to see how
repressed these dudes were. Their
own sexuality, not to mention the
sexuality of women, scared then to
death. Any wee amount of fun or
relaxation was so scary it led
directly to eternal damnation.
Demons and witches were everywhere
as they transferred their own
repressed desires onto the world
around them. Like all severely
repressed people they needed to lash
out at anyone a little bit freer.
Hell, they took on the hardships of
colonization because they thought
the Church of England was too
Catholic. They were sure as hell
going to tell everyone else they ran
into how to run their lives. What a
sad and lonely time to be alive.

Unfortunately, they're still here or at least their philosophical children are. Sometimes they're easy to see. Islamic countries wrapping their women up in bags. Communist China and its devotion to the state. But I'm more concerned with the American versions because that's where I live and write. The rest of the world can worry about itself because we have plenty of puritans right here at home.

This is absolutely not a left/right political issue. I loathe both parties and that way of looking at the world. (Don't get me started on politics. That will be a later book.) Puritans show up on BOTH sides of the political spectrum: theocrats and the poorly named "moral majority" on the right, smug mommies and silly hippies on the left. They hate each other but share the same repressive goal to fuck up your life. Let's explore each of the three appetites and help you understand their influence.

How they fuck up your diet - All religions have dietary restrictions and demands for their adherents. Jews and Moslems don't eat pork; many Buddhists are vegetarian; traditional Catholics never eat meat on Friday. The list

goes on and on. Most of those rules
possibly made sense at the time.
People didn't know about
trichinosis, ate undercooked pork
and died so the religious leaders
told them not to do that. Poor
monks rarely could afford meat so
they turned it into a virtue. If
you want to follow rules that were
relevant two thousand years ago, you
go right ahead. It's no skin off my
ass. But don't pretend that they're
actually relevant today. They
aren't. And don't pretend that they
make you more holy. They don't.
They make you anachronistic.

     The holiest holidays in many
religions, Lent, Passover, and
Ramadan, are defined by periods of
fasting and feasting. The beginning
of many spiritual journeys, be it
entering a monastery or starting a
vision quest, start with a cleansing
fast. Seems reasonable enough.
Clear the instrument in order to
prepare for the holy experience. I
don't disagree at all. I do it
pretty regularly myself. I even
start the diet in this book with a
modified fast. But it's a tool, not
a lifestyle. Just because short
term deprivation is useful DOESN'T
mean that long term deprivation is a
good idea. That's bad logic and a

bad lifestyle choice.

It's not just the religious types that want to tell you what to eat. I used to live in San Francisco and I can't spit without hitting a vegetarian. Ah yes, vegetarian; ancient Indian word for very bad hunter. There are a thousand arguments for vegetarianism and every single one of them is BULLSHIT. Humans are omnivores. We eat anything. Our bodies digest meat without any problem. Our eyes are in front of our heads because we're hunters, not prey. We need the amino acids and proteins in meat to thrive. Unfortunately none of these arguments make a single bit of difference because vegetarianism is a belief system, not a fact.

There, that's kind of the point. Don't let a belief system rule your diet. Use facts instead. God based diets or hippy love for fuzzy creatures are perfectly fine. It's a free country; believe any damn fool thing you want. Just don't pretend they're facts.

I'd also like to personally condemn the newest hippy bullshit movement, the fetish over local, organically grown food. What an arrogant, smug view of the world. Sure, eating only the highest

quality, locally grown food is great
if you happen to be rich and live in
California. Preaching your utopian
claptrap doesn't do anyone any good
and many of us know its true purpose
is to make them feel superior to
everybody else. The rest of the
world is poor and has winter so shut
the fuck up.

How they fuck up inebriation -
Puritans are repressed. That's how
they got to be puritans. In order
to stay repressed they need to keep
absolute control of themselves at
all times. They also have to make
sure that they're not tempted by
anything you might be doing.
Anything that might lead to fun
needs to be stopped immediately,
usually through laws. The examples
are so plentiful and obvious I'll
just make a quick list:

• Prohibition. How did that work
  out? But the anti-alcohol forces
  haven't really gone away. They
  raised the drinking age to 21.
  Sure that makes sense. You can
  vote, get married, and go to war
  but you can't have a beer when
  you get home. Really? Don't be
  fooled. Groups like Mothers
  Against Drunk Drivers might seem
  reasonable, but they're really
  just puritans with a new facade.

- No smoking. Tobacco is a perfectly legal product. So why can't I smoke in bars or at the park or 10,000 other places? I've got a news flash for you. There is not one shred of evidence that second hand smoke is a real problem. Puritans again.

- Marijuana - You and I both know lots of people who use it. I used to. So what? Why exactly is it illegal? Some puritans are so evil they actually want to keep it from AIDS and cancer patients who need it. And they represent God?

- The war against some drugs - What a crock of shit. It hasn't worked and it shouldn't. Why can the government tell you what you can put in your own damn body?

- Puritanism: The worry that someone, somewhere, is living a better life than you are. I guess they're right. We are. I could go on and on but I'd just get me more worked up and I'd have to get some whisky and this chapter would never get finished. I'm sure you've gotten the idea by now.

  How they fuck up sex - If you

think puritans are repressed around inebriation wait until you see what they do to sex. Ironically both the left and right use the same phrase to bludgeon their viewpoints into the public dialogue, "What about the children." Whenever I hear that phrase I know that I'm about to hear puritan bullshit. They've used shame, the FCC, the legitimate issue of child porn, and the fear of AIDS to scare people out of their own sexuality. Any amount of graphic violence is fine but a nipple on TV almost destroyed modern American society. Please please please read the chapter on sexuality even if it makes you uncomfortable. Don't let the puritans win and your joyful life lose.

Whenever I start to rant about this shit there's always some idiot who tells me to just relax, the puritans are concerned people and they aren't doing any real harm. I have two responses to that. First, you're wrong on a philosophical level. Every time they rob joy from someone's life the world is a little poorer place. Second, you're wrong on a physical level. A bunch of stupid puritan hippies have decided that vaccinations are unnecessary and dangerous. When people start

dying of smallpox or polio we'll see
if it does any real harm.

I know I tend to get a little
heated up on this subject. I find
it truly offensive. Puritans think
they know better than you do. They
don't. Or they think they know what
God wants. They don't. God might
be joy and love. Why would God want
you to let other people tell you
what to do if he created you? And
if you don't believe in God the
questions are even more profound.
Why do you let a society based in
the Judeo-Christian tradition
determine your behavior? And as if
this isn't bad enough, the puritans
allow themselves to be used by other
malevolent forces fuck you up. On
to the squirrels...

CHAPTER 5: EVIL SQUIRRELS & BULLSHIT

The new puritans are a problem but they aren't the only one. There's a whole legion of evil little squirrels looking to manipulate your appetites for their own gain. I couldn't begin to detail all of them even if I were writing an encyclopedia so you'll need to learn to ferret out the nasty little fuckers yourself. In the meantime, I'll give you a short list of some of the worst offenders...

Politics - Politicians are easily controlled by puritans. Why else are the taxes so high on cigarettes and alcohol? Half the damn laws they pass are to please the most repressed members of society. If they ever came out in favor of sex or inebriation the opposition would label them a pervert and chase them out of office. When is the last time you heard a politician espouse a non-Christian value?

Politicians also love to manipulate you by demonizing anything different. You probably wouldn't vote for him if you were paying attention to what he's actually doing so he scares you with someone else's sexuality or joyful overindulgence. Oldest trick in the book.

Commerce - We live in a capitalist society. Not that I'm complaining but it does have certain limitations. One of these is that people will lie to you to sell you shit. I know, not exactly a news flash. Nonetheless, a lot of what you think you know about appetites comes from media that makes its living by taking your money. Not exactly an uninterested source. So buyer beware. Always.

Doctors and drug companies - As I just noted, capitalism has some weak spots. The way we deal with health care is one of them. Would it surprise you that the companies that make cholesterol drugs have a huge hand in setting the guidelines for elevated cholesterol? It shouldn't. It's almost impossible to be too paranoid.

Media and body image - The people you see on television and in movies are beautiful to start with. On top of that they're covered in makeup and expensive clothes. After that they're shot through special lenses and Photoshopped to make them

look even better. But still we
think that we should aim to look
like that. Wrong. It will only
make you crazy.

The world hates ignorance -
Wanna know a secret? Nobody really
knows a whole lot about how humans
work or how to keep them healthy.
Everybody, and I mean EVERYBODY, is
guessing. How much should you
weigh? No one knows. How much
should you work out? Everybody's
guessing. Me too. That's why this
book is pretty basic. 'Cause I
don't feel the need to fill it full
of crap to make myself look smart.

It's your body. Find your own
information. Be skeptical. Trust
your instincts. And don't let
anyone else tell you what to do or
else we'll live in the world of
"Escape From LA." The United States
is a nonsmoking nation! No smoking,
drugs, alcohol, women - unless
you're married, foul language, or
red meat! Yeah sure, Land of the
Free.

CHAPTER 6: SOME REALISTIC FOOD ADVICE

So now you know how the
puritans, squirrels, and bullshit
are lined up against you. Before we
move on to the actual diet, I want
to make sure you have a few basic
food facts that everyone should
know, but few do. It includes
vitamins, diet tips, and other
useful crap. Even if you ignore the
rest of the diet stuff in this book
you should always consider the
following things:

- Changes in diet and lifestyle
  frequently lead to constipation.
  Just stress alone can do it too.
  Go to the drugstore and buy
  psyllium root capsules. Take 2
  every day, one with breakfast and
  one with dinner. They'll keep
  you nice and regular. Do it now.

- Eat meat. Eat red meat. You
  don't have to do it all the time.
  Two or three times a week is
  enough. Red meat includes amino
  acids and fats that your body
  needs.

- Take a multivitamin and an extra
  antioxidant every day. You can
  take other supplements if you

want, but at least take these two.

- Real food is always better for you than processed food. If it exists in nature, eat it. If it doesn't, avoid it. Roast beef and ham are better for you than bologna or hot dogs. Fried chicken is easier for your body to digest and use than chicken "nuggets." A little awareness can make a big difference.

- Fast food isn't evil, but it isn't wonderful either. Make it a treat rather than a staple.

- Caffeine is good. It gives you a higher metabolic rate and stimulates your nervous system. Spread it throughout the day rather than spikes in the morning for the best results.

- Drink lots of water and make it cold if you can. Just do it. Every day. It's the simplest thing you can do to be healthier.

- Eat a big breakfast. If you want a fat splurge, morning is the best time. If you ingest a lot of your calories in the morning you'll gain less weight over time and it keeps your metabolism higher all day.

- Don't eat right before bed. It's

inefficient and hard on your body. At least two to three hours between dinner and bedtime is the minimum.

- Don't skimp on the dairy. It's good for you and helps you digest fat.

- Choose low-fat when it doesn't matter. For the life of me, I can't tell the difference between low fat sour cream or cream cheese and their full fat counterparts. So why the hell not?

- Exercise. Use heavier weights and do your cardio. If you don't know how, go buy my book "Get Off Your Ass."

- Relax and get centered. The less stress you have the more efficiently your body works. If you need help go buy my book "Inner Workout Fu." Okay, enough shameless plugging. On to the reality of genetics.

CHAPTER 7: THE REALITY OF GENETICS

I'm sure you've heard the Irish prayer that says, God grant me the courage to change the things I can, the patience to accept the things I can't, and the wisdom to know the difference. Most of my books are about changing the things you can. This chapter and the next are about accepting the things you can't. No matter how committed and disciplined you might be there are two things that you just can't change: genetics and time.

You are who you are. To some extent your genetics are your destiny. Your height, bone structure, body type, and perhaps life span are determined by your DNA. You got to dance with what brung ya. No amount of exercising and diet is going to make me any taller or give me a larger penis. Similarly the healthiest diet in the world won't make me any younger. If you think otherwise you're either a fool or you've fallen under the spell of malevolent squirrels.

Look, I don't know you and I'm not your doctor. I don't even play one on TV. I'm in no position to

tell you how much you should weigh
and neither is anyone else. Your
body might shed pounds easily and
keep them off with minimal effort.
Or it might hold on to every ounce
even if you live on celery and
water. I can tell you that a good
diet will give you an overall
healthier look. Your skin should be
clear, your hair shinier, and your
nails thicker. It should also give
you more energy during the day and
more libido at night since your
system is working with more
efficiency. But I can't tell you
how hard it will be. Only your
genetics know that.

Remember how, during your teens
and twenties you could eat
practically anything and not gain a
pound? When you're hovering around
middle age you'll probably find
that's just won't be the case
anymore. Metabolism naturally slows
down as we age so weight gain creeps
up on us as we head through our
thirties. You also naturally lose
muscle mass past thirty unless you
do something to counteract it. Time
marches on and we age right along
with it. Besides, there are worse
things than being fat.

I know obesity is a huge
problem and shouldn't be

underestimated. However there needs
to be a clear distinction between
"overweight" and "not shaped like a
20 year old model" A 50 year old
woman who looks like Paris Hilton is
more than a little tragic. As we
get older we should be developing
the skills of wisdom and compassion
and this growth should be reflected
in our bodies. The areas for wisdom
and power are from your heart chakra
to your hara, two inches below your
belly button. Aging allows
development of "center" and the
ability to be "centered." We should
glory in the physical manifestation
of this work even if it's going to
mean a little thickness around the
middle. We would all do well to
remember that War Gods are lean and
Buddha is always a little "thick
around the middle."

I'm not trying to discourage
you. Huge change is possible.
Anyone can get leaner, stronger,
healthier, and more in control.
Even if genetics do determine life
span you can add a lot of quality to
those last years if you're in shape.
I just don't want you to think
miracles are going to happen.
That's why we do an intellectual
diet before we do a physical one...

CHAPTER 8: INTELLECTUAL CLEANSING

One of my favorite Zen stories involves the prerequisite to learning. An advanced student wanted to study with a very famous teacher but every time he requested a position the old master declined to accept him. After a few years the student demanded to know why and the teacher invited him to tea. When the student extended his cup, the master filled it with hot tea but didn't stop at the top. He just kept pouring and the hot tea went all over the table and dripped onto the student's lap. The student jumped up and called the master a fool. When he'd calmed down the master explained that the student was the teacup, already so full of knowledge that he couldn't learn anything new. If he wanted to be his student, he'd have to empty his cup first. That's the purpose of this chapter. A brain diet before the body diet.

Hopefully you've already discarded all of the puritan and evil squirrel bullshit. Now let's get rid of some other crap that's collected in our psyche. Like guilt

and recriminations. And time
expectations. And ego bullshit.
And oh yeah, body image.

There are three basic body
types: ectomorph, endomorph, and
mesomorph; also known as fat,
skinny, and lucky. It's a simple
fact of human life that everybody
wants to be something they aren't.
Comedians want to be rock stars
while rock stars want to be artists,
artists want to be actors and actors
want to be comedians. This is
especially true of body types. Fat
people want to be thin, skinny
people want to bulk up and everyone
wants to be a muscle bound
mesomorph. Too bad. Remember the
last chapter? Good. Accept and
love your own body type. It's not
like you have a choice.

As long as you're accepting
things you might as well get
comfortable with where you are in
the process. However you got here
is irrelevant. I don't care what
you did yesterday or last week or
last year. There are only two time
frames that matter: today and next
year. Are you doing everything you
can do today and will you still be
doing it next year. Nothing else
matters.

Before you go on to the next

chapter do two more things. First,
commit to a brain fast. You're
going to clean out your system and I
think it helps to clean out your
mind first. Before you start
dieting take a couple of days and
relax. Go to the beach or the
mountains if you can. Take some
long walks and some quiet sits.
Turn off the television and let any
news from the outside world take
care of itself. No newspapers or
internet. And no working. Two days
of peace and quiet as a brain enema.

Secondly, decide if your goals
include weight loss. They might
not. They might just include
control, power, a healthier body,
and more joy. If so, good for you
and skip the rest of this chapter.
If you do want to lose weight give
some thought to how much and keep
reading.

Go get on a scale. I know
getting on a scale can be really
traumatic because we attach all
sorts of ego issues to that bullshit
number. Hell, some people define
themselves and their value as human
beings to the number that comes up.
This won't help. It's just a number
and nothing more and its only value
is comparative. Try to detach from
any other feelings that come up when

it's time to weigh in. Weigh in
once a week. Your weight fluctuates
wildly during the week and can make
you crazy if you track it too
closely. Once a week is plenty.
Always weigh in at the same time, on
the same day. This will ensure a
more realistic comparison. Also try
to use the same scale every time.
Remember, don't get attached to the
number. It is simply data and has
no other meaning.

Always keep in mind that the
time you spend losing weight is
temporary. The restrictive, lower
calorie regime only lasts as long as
you want it to. After that comes
maintenance and that's way easier
because you no longer have to run at
a deficit.

After you hit your target
weight you'll need to set a trigger
number. This trigger should be a
round number a few pounds heavier
than your target weight. For
example, if you got down to 130
pounds, you'd set your trigger
number at 140. Continue your weekly
weigh in at the same time and in the
same way as you had been during your
weight loss process. As long as
your weekly weigh in is below your
trigger number, you don't need to do
anything. If your weigh in is over

your target number, you'll just have
to go back to your good foods and
cut out your sensitive foods for a
couple of weeks.

CHAPTER 9:
BATTLING EGO

Your ego is not your friend.
In fact it's probably going to do
everything it can to fuck you up.
Your ego hates change even if that
change is for the positive. What is
your ego? It's a set of
assumptions, fears, self-deceptions,
and self-conceits. Sure it has its
purpose but that purpose is all too
often to keep you from changing.
Your ego wants nothing more than to
protect itself from feeling stupid
or powerless or at risk.

Your ego is going to tell you
all kinds of shit. Here's how to
deal with the evil little fucker.
Take a few minutes once a week and
get into a really good mental space.
Use your sacred space (see book 1)
or your meditations (see book 3).
When you're happy and calm, make
decisions about what you can do
during the next week. Set up your
priorities and REFUSE TO CHANGE
THEM. You make good decisions while
you're in a centered state. Any
decision you make to change it is
bound to be worse and is most likely
your ego.

Unlike ego, endorphins ARE your

friend. Endorphins are these magic
little fuckers that your brain
releases under certain
circumstances. They kill pain and
make you feel good about yourself.
If Joy is a chemical endorphins are
it. They're released during sex,
when you drink alcohol or eat
chocolate, etc. But your brain
doesn't want you running around in a
state of perpetual bliss so it also
releases endorphin killers after an
endorphin spike. Therefore if you
eat chocolate constantly or drink
too much every day the endorphin
killers begin to dominate and you
feel like shit.

Keeping a constant level of
endorphins will keep you in a good
mood and we both know that you'll
make better decisions. One of the
tricks to higher endorphin levels is
exercise. So go do some.

Another way to manipulate
endorphins is to use music. Music,
especially loud music, jacks up
endorphins. So if you feel you need
a little help put on the headphones
and crank it up. Okay, enough
preparation. Here we go on to the
diet...

CHAPTER 10: PHYSICAL CLEANSING

Well, we're finally here. The diet part. The word "diet" means all the food that you consume during a given period of time. You're on a diet now. It might consist of nothing but fast food, pizza, and cookies but it is a diet. In some ways all diets are dictated. Availability, cultural norms, seasons, taste, income level, and a thousand other things effect what makes up your diet. In our culture "diet" has come to mean an artificial dictate to eat certain foods while avoiding other ones. Since this is ultimately arbitrary it's no surprise that "diets" don't work for most people.

Your diet should do two things: provide for your body's health and bring you moments of joy and pleasure. The first goal will be accomplished by starting you out with a short fast to cleanse your system. We'll follow that with a series of personal experiments to find the foods that make your body run efficiently. The results of this study can be combined with the facts from chapter six to give you your healthy choices.

There's a public perception that overweight people just lack will power. Nothing could be further from the truth. Judging by how long some dieters wait to eat and the things that they'll deny themselves obese people have extraordinary willpower. However using this willpower to avoid eating while hungry is both counterproductive to your diet and stupid. Using willpower to deny yourself food will only lead you to pile on more pounds and make you miserable. If you restrict your food intake your body goes for too long without an energy source and it responds by temporarily slowing your metabolism. When you finally eat your body responds by hoarding calories and urging you to consume more food than your body can burn to guard against the next starvation cycle. That's not helpful or healthy. Don't mess around with this powerful internal energy shutoff mechanism. In short, don't get hungry.

Hunger works against you in another way, too. By the time you salivate you're much more interested in a quick energy fix like sugar than a healthier alternative so you're less likely to make good choices. Weight loss isn't brain surgery. Making sure your system is efficient will take you a long way, but if you want to lose a lot of weight you need to take in fewer calories than you burn. Okay, let's get started.

- The first step on your diet path is clean out your body. We're going to do this with a five day modified fast. This is necessary for a lot of reasons:

- It provides a break in your routine that will allow you to set new patterns at the start of your new life.

- It cleans out the junk that has collected in your system over the years.

- Once your system is cleaner your responses to food will be exaggerated and allow you to collect good data about yourself

- Any dependencies on food that you have will be broken.

- You can notice any cravings that come up and give you even more information.

- It'll jump-start your metabolism.

- You'll drop a few pounds quickly to provide a little momentum.

This isn't a starve yourself fast, it just limits the foods you eat for a short period of time. Don't panic! It won't be as hard as you think it will and it'll be over before you know it. You can eat all you want, just not what you want. Here are the rules:

- Stay on the fast for 5 full days.
- Don't cheat at all.
- Drink lots of water.
- Don't take any nonprescription drugs or vitamins.
- Don't chew gum.
- Go for a walk every day.

Here's a list of ALL the foods you're allowed to eat during the five days of your cleansing fast. Remember that you shouldn't eat ANYTHING that's not on the list. This includes things you might use during preparation of other ingredients.

- Rice, any kind
- Chicken
- Carrots
- Green beans
- Cucumbers
- Lettuce, any standard variety
- Olive oil
- Salt

- Water

After the five days of your cleansing fast are over you can begin the process that will lead to your personal diet. You're going to use your body and its reactions as a science experiment. The fast has cleaned your system out so you're reactions to foods will be exaggerated. Every time you introduce a new food you'll be able to easily judge whether it has a positive or negative effect on your body chemistry.

Everyone's body chemistry is unique. Your digestive process is made up a huge combination of enzymes, hormones, and various biotic cultures that have taken up residence in your intestines. This means that your system will have its own strengths and weaknesses. Sometimes the weaknesses of your system are referred to as allergies or intolerances, as in "I'm allergic to seafood" or "I'm lactose intolerant." These characterizations carry with them an underlying value judgment that implies there is something wrong with you or you're lacking in some way.

It's important to abandon this

idea. Everyone has foods that their
system do well with and foods that
they struggle to digest. No one's
system is any "better" than anyone
else's. Here are the guidelines for
adding foods back to your daily
diet:

- Add any foods you'd like, in any
  order.

- Only add one food per day. Don't
  add foods in combination with
  each other. When you try each
  food, try it by itself.

- When you react badly to
  something, go back to all safe
  foods the next day and don't try
  anything new until the following
  day.

- Treat each food as unique. You
  might be fine with cheese but
  have trouble drinking milk. They
  should be tried separately even
  though they're both dairy.

- Lunch is the best meal to try new
  foods since you'll have all
  afternoon to look for reactions.

- There are some foods that very
  few   people react badly to.
  They can usually be added quickly
  with a minimum of side effects.
  They are: beef and pork, corn and
  corn products, most oils (not
  peanut), most vegetables, turkey

and other fowl, and potatoes.
- The following is a list of foods
  that a lot of people find that
  they have trouble with. You
  should be extra vigilant when you
  add them to your diet: wheat,
  yeast, soy, dairy, peanuts,
  tomatoes, fruit and citrus, and
  beans.

After you add each new food
you're looking for three very
specific things: bloating,
gastrointestinal distress, or an
energy crash. Each of these are
explained specifically below. Be
alert for these symptoms in the few
hours after the meal and the next
morning. If they show up then you
know that this is not a food that
your system deals with well. If you
feel great afterward, it's a food
that your system likes. Couldn't be
simpler.

BLOATING - If your body is
having trouble digesting something
it produces gas. This gas will make
you feel heavy or fat. You'll also
get very thirsty since you'll be
retaining water. While this is a
little hard to explain the first
time it happens, you'll recognize it
immediately. It will usually occur
1-4 hours after you try the new
food.

GI DISTRESS - This is the
easiest thing to recognize since
it's typified by multiple rapid
trips to the bathroom. When your
system is given something that it
doesn't deal well with it'll
immediately try to get rid of
everything in the pipeline very
quickly, usually in the form of
diarrhea. This might occur anytime
after the new food, or even after
the next meal or the next morning.

ENERGY - This is the subtlest
but most important sign. Food is
ultimately an energy source for your
body. If something is hard for you
to digest it'll take up energy
rather than supply it. You should
feel good after a meal. If you feel
sleepy or draggy after lunch than
something in your lunch is messing
up the system. This is the surest
sign that it's not a good food for
you.

As you add more and more foods
you'll need to keep some lists in
order to track your data. This
might seem like a lot of work but it
really isn't that hard. Remember,
you'll have these answers for the
rest of your life! Once you have
your personal data, you have the
basis for your long-term diet. This
list is just data. It doesn't mean

don't eat the foods on your
sensitive list, just know that
you'll pay a price for doing so. It
also means that these foods are
counterproductive to weight loss
since they make your system less
efficient. If you're trying to lose
weight, try not to eat them. Just
avoiding these foods will make your
body shed weight pretty quickly.
It'll also guarantee that as long as
you keep these foods in their place,
you'll never gain weight again. If
you want to lose a lot of weight, or
lose it more quickly, you'll have to
cut your calories. There is no
other way.

Use the new information to take
control of your diet. Good, now
we're ready to drink and get stoned…

CHAPTER 11: DRUGS, ALCOHOL & TOBACCO

There is no such thing as "demon rum," there is only rum. There is no drug scourge and nothing to be at war against, there are only a few substances that humans take in order to make themselves feel a little better, a little worse, or just different. They aren't good or evil; they just simply are. As a society we never deal with inebriates realistically and it's much to our own detriment. Real education and decision making would make everybody happier.

The puritan squirrels will tell you there is no good reason to take drugs or get drunk. You know that's wrong. I know it's wrong. Hell, they might even know it's wrong. So let's just leave them to their sad little existence and look at some of the reasons why inebriates are good:

* Many inebriates are pleasurable. There, I said it. Pleasure pleasure pleasure. Can't you just see the little fuckers cringing? Pleasure is GOOD. Pleasure is HEALTHY. Pleasure is JOYFUL and HOLY. Having a few

drinks or a couple of tokes feels
great. That's reason enough.
     * Inebriates add fun. They can
make dull times good and good times
great. There is NOTHING wrong with
having a little fun. Or a lot.
     * Sometimes things really suck.
People die. Relationships end.
Catastrophe strikes. Using as
inebriate as a short term tool is a
damn good idea. Unless you like
suffering.
     * Stress relief. Stress isn't
inherently bad for you. Too much
stress is. Inebriates can offer a
short vacation and quick recharge of
the batteries.
     * Sometimes we get too stuck in
our heads or trapped within our own
experiences and perceptions.
Inebriates can offer mind expanding
opportunities.
     * Let's face it, sometimes we
get stuck in our own inhibitions. A
little lubrication is exactly what
you need. They also give us the
excuse to do what we wanted to do
anyway but couldn't quite give
ourselves permission. That's why
girls like to have a little too much
to drink. It allows them to explain
away why they did what they really
wanted to...
     * It's not a coincidence that

many great artists, musicians, and writers were also great drinkers or drug takers. They can really help with the creative process. Of course they can also kill you.

Don't get me wrong. I know how dangerous these substances can become when they aren't controlled. But that control has to be personal, not legal or religious. The whole point of this book is to give you control and allow to make choices. Addiction takes all that away from you. An addict has no control, no freedom, and doesn't get to make many choices for themselves. But that risk is no excuse to ignore or just live without the positive attributes.

Inebriates are exactly like food in this way. Being a fat pig will kill you and rob you of your freedom but never eating a bacon cheeseburger is just stupid. The specter of addiction means that making bad drug choices has really serious consequences. The mistake is in thinking that "just saying no" doesn't have equally bad consequences. Same with sex too. That's why equate them as appetites. So let's have some good drug info...

Alcohol - Nothing wrong with having a drink, or eight. Beer, wine, and spirits are great in reasonable amounts. I prefer Scotch. Here are my thoughts

- Don't drink and drive. Duh.
- Don't drink every day. Make conscious choices about when and where.
- Don't drink to avoid problems. It won't help.
- Learn how much you can handle. There's nothing worse than some drunken college idiot passing out or throwing up. A little experience and self-awareness can add up to a lot of class.
- Understand that being drunk in public can mean being a victim.

Tobacco - The problem with tobacco is that its addictive qualities make you use too much of it. A few cigars or cigarettes every couple of months is fine. Two packs a day will kill you. If you can't smoke occasionally, don't smoke at all.

Marijuana - A lot like tobacco in that smoking every day must be bad for you. Otherwise I'm a big fan. Relaxing, fun and if you use it sparingly you can stay pretty productive. I try to limit to a couple times a week. That seems pretty reasonable. Oh, and don't get arrested.

Sugar - Surprised to see that one here, aren't you? It's a drug all right. Creates euphoria and addiction. Treat it like a benign drug and limit it just like you would with any other inebriate.

Caffeine - Another drug that I like a lot in moderation. And by moderation I mean two or three hits a day. Go for it, just stop by 4:00 or so unless you want your sleep fucked up.

Hallucinogens - Use with caution. They might reveal things you aren't ready to know yet. They will enrich your life though. Just be sure to use a little common sense. Occasionally is plenty and always have a minder who'll stay straight and help out if things go badly.

Heavily 'addictive' drugs - Cocaine, heroin, meth, etc. Personally, I mostly stay away. Who needs the hassle of heavy addiction and withdrawal. But that's just me.

I'd like to finish this chapter with a special note to killjoy mommies and repressed theocrats. Yes, I just spent an entire chapter advising people to get use some drugs, get stoned, and get drunk occasionally. And I meant it. My

father was an alcoholic and cocaine
addict who probably died of an
overdose. I know all about
addiction. I know all about
bullshit too. And "just say no" is
bullshit. So fuck you. In Vino
Veritas.

CHAPTER 12: SEX AND SEXUALITY

Why is it that we're so incredibly uncomfortable with bodily functions? We urinate and defecate every single day and yet most people get twitchy as soon as you mention it. Most of our profanity is bodily function based. It makes no sense and frankly I just don't get it. And if you mention sexual function or genitals, it gets even worse. Damn, we're a fucked up species.

I know deep in my heart that a big percentage of my readers will skip this chapter. Some of you will read it but pretend they didn't. Nearly everyone will blush or squirm a little. And that's EXACTLY THE PROBLEM.

I'm male. I have a penis. Nearly half the world has one too. The other half has vaginas. It's not like either of them is particularly rare or exceptional but just try putting one on television. Anyone in this society who appears to be overtly sexual is shamed off the public stage while we download tons of porn. (It's not a coincidence that Utah, our most religious and repressed state, also leads the nation in amount of porn downloaded.) But just because our society is hypocritical and full of shit doesn't mean you have to be.

Sex is one of our most basic instincts, second only to food and shelter. Our DNA wants to replicate itself and it wants to do it really badly. It doesn't matter whether you believe in God, evolution, or space monkeys, that simple fact still exists. Who started it is a discussion for another time. In order to ensure that we'll reproduce, our DNA does two things: it makes sex really pleasurable and gives us a tremendous drive to go find it. Okay. Makes sense. So why do we keep trying to second guess nature or genes or God? If we can eat when we're hungry because we need food to live why can't we fuck when we're horny 'cause we need sex to live?

Don't say it. Don't even think it. We DO need sex. Sure, it's possible to live without it. It's possible to live on almost no food, too. That doesn't mean it's a good healthy idea. Getting control of your appetites means coming to terms with your own sexuality. Unfortunately that also means learning to live with a lot of

social disapproval. We don't live
in the best of all possible worlds.
     It all starts with
masturbation. If you don't
masturbate you need to start right
now. Do whatever you have to do in
order to get past whatever repressed
garbage is holding you up. For the
rest of you, you know you do it.
Quit lying to yourself and others.
Masturbation is good. Masturbation
is healthy both physically and
psychologically. It feels good and
teaches us about our own likes and
dislikes. Yet who but the boldest
amongst us can talk about it?
Nonetheless, masturbate more.
     While you're pleasuring
yourself be sure to let your
fantasies run wild. Fantasy and
imagination let us try different
things without risk. Use fantasy to
figure out what kinds of sex you
might like. If something really
turns you on in a fantasy you might
want to try it in real life. By
using this tool you can eventually
become aware of your own personal
sexuality. And that's a good thing.
More choice and more control.
     At this point I should probably
give my definition of good sex:
anything between consenting adults
that brings pleasure or fulfillment

to everyone involved. Period. And
I said adults. If you molest
children you're beneath contempt.
Get healed or get dead. I said
consenting, too. If you want to
rape women I hope the one you pick
is well trained and armed to the
teeth because the world will be a
way better when you're gone. I'm
not kidding. In my self defense
book I advise rape victims to kill
their attackers if possible.

     As far as I'm concerned rape
and child molestation are the only
two things off limits. There are
probably as many fetishes as there
are people. Most sexual morals are
nothing more than passing fads.
Ankles were hot in 1890. Now, not
so much. If you like it find a
willing partner and do it. S & M,
bondage, role play, oral, anal,
whatever. I'm sure you can find all
the possibilities you ever imagined
online. And what's more, be
comfortable and proud of your
tastes. I like pot stickers. I
like blow jobs too. So what.

     A quick word here on monogamy.
Yes, it's the norm, but what does it
really mean? Everyone has the right
to define that for themselves. Is
watching porn cheating? How about
virtual sex? How about a deep

emotional relationship that doesn't involve sex? Or vice versa? Make sure you and your actual or potential partner have the same definition or somebody's gonna get hurt. And non-monogamous relationships are really cool, too. I really want a girlfriend and my wife knows it. Whatever floats your boat.

We MUST stop being so sexually judgmental as a people. It's tearing us apart. I've written that the whole anti-gay marriage movement is sex based. If a man's wife died and his male friend moved in to help him raise his kids everyone would think that was heroic. If those same two men start kissing, everyone has a fit. Stop it. If you get comfortable with your own sexual appetite you'll probably be a lot less concerned with those of your neighbors.

CHAPTER 13: JOY TO THE WORLD

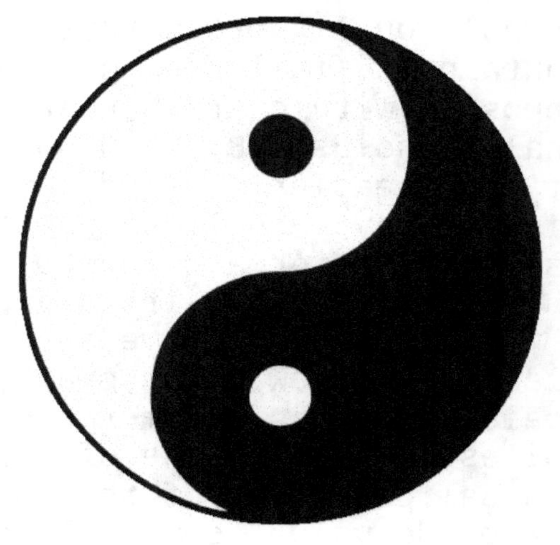

I'm sure you're familiar with
the yin yang symbol. If not, I
included one right here. I don't
want to get too philosophical (I'll
leave that to a later book) but
everything in the universe exists as
a duality. Black and white, tall
and short, you get the idea. I
believe that in order to gain
control of your life you need to
understand and control your
appetites. The thesis I've
presented in this book is that the
best way to do that is to master the
balance between joyful indulgence
and healthy restraint.

When you look at the yin yang

symbol you'll notice that each color
contains a small drop of it's
opposite within its borders. The
analogy holds. By being healthy
it'll be easier to find joy and by
finding joy, you'll be healthier.
As you move forward try to remember
this image and use it as a guide.

Let eating become a true
pleasure. Slow down, plan your
meals, and enjoy them to their
fullest. Food is one of the great
sensual pleasures of the world. Use
it to add value to your life.
Become comfortable with your
sexuality and let it be displayed
freely. Use the tool of inebriation
to relax, let go, and have fun
without it destroying your
usefulness as a human being.

A Taoist monk once said that
the secret to enlightenment is to
eat when you're hungry and sleep
when you're tired. He's probably
right but if you think about it
you'll realize how hard this dictum
really is. It's impossibly easy to
become distracted and forget your
priorities. The best intentions are
useless if you forget them during
your hectic day. Use my other books
to help you keep on the straight and
narrow. Morihei Ueshiba was right.
The true path is paper thin and one

paper's width is no longer the way.
So go forth and find both joy and
health. Vaya con Dios and Viva la
Revolucion!

<u>DIET NOTES:</u>

DIET NOTES:

DIET NOTES:

<u>DIET NOTES:</u>

DIET NOTES:

<u>DIET NOTES:</u>

DIET NOTES:

<u>DIET NOTES:</u>

<u>DIET NOTES:</u>

<u>DIET NOTES:</u>

ONE FINAL NOTE

You are a unique individual. You and you alone, are ultimately responsible for your actions. Just about everything in the Testaments of the Temple of the Circus Monkey is the expressed opinion of Laird Archbishop Angus McIntosh. He thinks they're right and he thinks they'll help you live a fuller, funner life. However, results are clearly not guaranteed. Doing anything active carries risk and that risk is all yours. So don't sue me. You have been warned.

Badass Canes

The Badass Cane - A strong, 36 inch long, 3/4 inch thick hickory cane that's been modified for better use as a weapon. The crook has been cut down, the hand grip's been extended, and a heavyweight ferrule is placed on the bottom. And it's painted black, cause black is cool. There is nothing that will keep this cane from going through metal detectors or keep it from qualifying as a necessary disabled appliance. Every Badass Cane package comes complete with cane, a spare heavy duty ferrule, and a copy of The Badass Cane book to explain your rights and help you use it efficiently.

Clothing

Look great while being a little cheeky in our line of T-shirts, tank tops, and sweatshirts.

Available at KWChop.com

More Books

Angus has written a lot more stuff. TCM Publishing also has books by other authors. Come check it out.

Unweapons Accessories

The ultimate Unweapons are everyday items that you have on your person when you need them and that you won't get stopped and hassled for having. Check out our line of self protection secret weapon necklaces, bracelets, and keychains that you can wear in plain sight. Plus, they're awesome and fabulous to add to any outfit!

Packages

Along with the BadAss Cane package, we offer many more for great deals. Come check them out!

Available at KWChop.com

Desert Monkey Dojo and the Digital Dojo

Desert Monkey Dojo is serious training for less than serious people. We're a martial arts type school catering to students who are more interested in self improvement than violence, sport, or trophies. Our classes are small, intimate, intense, and fun. We believe in training hard but always with a sense of Joy.

DMD offers a variety of seminars and training.

We also have a Digital Dojo where you can learn in the comfort of your own home!

Find us at CircusMonkeyTemple.org & DesertMonkeyDojo.org

THE

END